Well in Twelve

How I Reversed Blindness and an Autoimmune Diagnosis
in Twelve Days

Alycea K. Shirley

Contents

I dedicate this book to my three lovely daughters; Tiwa, Iman, and Boatemaa. If it weren't for the three of you, I wouldn't have the strength, perseverance, or endurance to fight for my life and to write this book. I also dedicate this book to the millions of Americans suffering from Multiple Sclerosis and other forms of Autoimmune Disease, hoping my story can help bring you some resolve.

Introduction

I would like to start by saying, I am in no shape or form a doctor. I am rather a mother of three beautiful girls and a licensed Massage Therapist. I have always had an interest in holistic healing and alternative therapies. I have traveled, studied, and even practiced many therapies in search of answers to holistic health. But honestly, I didn't practice everything I learned. Some things I kept in the back of my mind not knowing one day it would save my life as they are the primary and most vital building structures to holistic health.

Chapter 1
Autoimmune Disease

Multiple Sclerosis, also known as MS, is a debilitating condition. The cause is currently unknown. It's considered an immune-mediated disease or autoimmune disease in which the body's immune system attacks its own tissues. In the case of MS, this immune system malfunction destroys the fatty substance that coats and protects nerve fibers in the brain and spinal cord (myelin). MS currently affects 2.5 million people around the globe, and in America, 200 new cases are diagnosed every week. It is most prevalent in young adults and in women.

It has many symptoms including: vision loss, pain in the back of eyes when you nod your head or with eye movement, blurred vision or double vision. Tremor can occur during precise movements in the hands or limbs. Muscular cramping, difficulty walking, inability to rapidly change motions, involuntary movements, muscle paralysis, muscle rigidity, muscle weakness, problems with coordination, stiff muscles, clumsiness, muscle spasms, or overactive reflexes. Whole body fatigue, dizziness, heat intolerance, poor balance, or vertigo are also symptoms of MS.

To make matters worse, there are side-lining issues that accompany the symptoms of MS. These issues include: Sensory issues such as the feeling of pins and needles, abnormality of taste, reduced sensation of touch, or uncomfortable tingling and burning. There are bladder issues including: excessive urination at night, leaking of urine, persistent urge to urinate, or urinary retention. Sexual issues of multiple sclerosis include erectile dysfunction or sexual dysfunction. You can have anxiety or mood swings. You may notice difficulty speaking or slurred speech.

Last but not least, other symptoms include: cognitive deficit, constipation, depression, difficulty swallowing, foot drop, headache, heavy legs, numbness of face, nystagmus, sleep deprivation, tongue numbness, or weakness. I had many of these symptoms but just shrugged them off to tiredness from work or thinking maybe "that's just how I am." But what made me decide to move forward with a lifestyle change was my sudden loss of vision.

Chapter 2
My Story

When I think about my story as it pertains to vision loss, I name it "The Day I Woke Up with a Dot in My Eye". It was a dot gray in color and somewhat blurry. It was in the center of my vision and only was in my left eye. Not only did I have a little gray dot but it was also accompanied by a severe headache on the left side of my head from the front to the back. Most of the pain was towards the front and especially when I moved my left eye about.

I was working as an outdoor salesman at the time during the summer in New Jersey, which was very hot, so I associated it with the extreme heat I was walking in all day. At this time I only had a one-year-old, and I was her sole provider. So, I had to go to work despite my pains. Also, the relationship I had with her father was very violent and volatile. It was causing me an immense amount of stress.

When I came home that day from work, as I walked through the door, he started to shout at me for what reason I can't remember at this time. But what I do remember is the pain that radiated from my eye every time he shouted. It felt as if I was going to die. I decided I would not engage in any more shouting matches with him from that day going forward because I realized my health was at stake. As the night went on and the shouting continued, the pain gradually increased.

The next day I woke up, hoping the headache would be gone, but it was even more severe, and this time the little gray dot was just a little bigger than the day before. I decided no matter what, I had to stay home from work that day. So, I stayed home and rested, hoping being out of the sun would help me. The father of my first child tried to provoke me with arguments, but I refused to engage. Instead, I used the time to lay down and meditate. Going to sleep that night, the pain was excruciating. All I could think about was my daughter and who would raise her if I died in my sleep.

The next day I decided I had to see a doctor. The little gray dot was bigger than before and covered most of the vision in my left eye. Firstly, I went to an ophthalmologist and told him everything that happened and what I was experiencing. He gave me an eye exam which confirmed that at this time I was legally blind in my left eye. During the test he had me look through a lens and I was to tell him if I saw a green light or not. When I was unable to confirm that I saw the green light, he then confirmed that I was legally blind in my left eye.

He looked into my eye and was also able to confirm that there was nothing actually wrong with my eye so it must have been the optical nerve that was the problem. He told me I needed to see a general doctor immediately. I then went to a medical doctor not too far from where I lived. I told her about the pain I was having and the story of the little gray dot. This time the dot was not so little. It was the third day and it had grown to cover most of the center of my eye. She told me she had to perform an MRI and I would have to come back three weeks later for the results. Three weeks? I panicked! With this pain I was sure I would've been dead in just a few days.

Remember when I told you I used to spend a lot of my time researching holistic health in the introduction? Well, during my self-studies, I learned about a man named Dr. Sebi. He was an herbal doctor, who was said to have cured HIV/AIDS and was summoned to court by the state of New York for his claims, as he wasn't an actual medical doctor and his claims were "unfounded". But surprisingly, he won. This intrigued me and I started to follow up with his findings for years.

His method to curing HIV/AIDS was an alkaline diet. Not only did he claim to cure HIV/AIDS, but a litany of other ailments and diseases. He actually claimed he could cure any disease with his method. I found this very interesting, but also kept it at the back of my mind, because in order to do a complete alkaline diet you must adhere to a strict and limited vegan diet. I wasn't ready. I loved my meat, cheese, and gluten too much! Even some of my favorite vegetables were restricted. So, although intrigued, I never committed.

I also had an aunt who was diagnosed with a brain tumor but no doctor could figure out a cure for her and it was devastating her life. She saw an herbal doctor who told her to fast for 40 days with a strict liquid diet consisting of blended and juiced fruits and vegetables. When she went back to the doctors, they couldn't find her tumor. They considered it a medical miracle. I decided to ask her for that doctor's number, as Dr. Sebi, who I studied for years, died the year before. She gave me his number and I immediately gave him a call and was scheduled to see him the very next day.

I went to see him and it was by chance and my luck that I was able to because he was a traveling doctor who traveled the 50 states month by month and he happened to be in my state that particular month and was leaving the very next week. Before I saw him he made me sign a contract stating that I would not give him up to local or federal authorities, because he practiced medicine that didn't adhere to their standards or beliefs. I was desperate and the medical doctors that I went to were not helping me or not helping urgently enough. So, I obliged. No, I won't give his full name, but I'll just call him Dr. C.

Dr. C literally saved my life. He too promoted veganism. The method he used to diagnose me was an eye exam, but it was no regular eye exam. He took a picture of my eye, amplified the picture and then read it based on each mark and indentation in my eye. Based off of his reading, he was able to tell me that I was pre-diabetic and that I had an onset of multiple sclerosis. He also told me that the left side of my brain was swollen and inflamed and this was causing the left eye to go blind.

I was frightened and afraid and asked him did I need to be worried. He looked me square in the eye and said "Absolutely, you are blind. Isn't that a cause for concern?". Feeling silly, but nonetheless determined to live, I asked him what I needed to do. He told me I needed to change my diet immediately, go vegan, remove certain oils out of my diet and take some supplements to help cleanse and fortify my body. He said I could buy the supplements on my own or I could buy them from him, the choice was mine.

Out of convenience and time constraints I decided I ought to buy them from him. He also helped me out so much and charged so little for his service, $70 for the assessment and consultation, I wanted to further support his cause. He then gave me a nutritional guide and sent me home. I was given a basic vegan diet from Dr. C, but I decided to also apply Dr. Sebi's alkaline vegan diet. I also used the supplements he gave me, and within days I started to feel the results.

After two days of eating clean, my headache dissipated completely and my vision improved day by day as well. Two weeks later I had an appointment with the ophthalmologist and after the vision test was performed he realized my vision had improved by 95%! He was astounded and asked how did I do it? When I said I stopped eating meat and changed my diet he laughed and said no way. I left smiling knowing the truth to my story.

I also went back to the medical doctor to get my MRI results. She confirmed to me based off the MRI results that I indeed had an onset of multiple sclerosis and the optical nerve of the left eye was inflamed which was the cause of my blindness. Now, for your information, the optical nerve is one of twelve cranial nerves. They are nerve pairs that are connected to your brain. This also confirmed what Dr. C said to me about the left side of my brain being inflamed.

I was still amazed at his work because he was able to diagnose me merely by looking into my eyes and gave me immediate results, compared to the MRI, a machine, which also included an injection of ink into my body for contrast, and I had to wait weeks for the results. This made me marvel at the wondrous work of man vs. machine and even more so at the holistic and natural way to healing your body vs. the medical approach.

She gave me a list of medications, including cortical steroids, that I needed to take immediately. She also told me that because of the litany of medication I would have to stop breast-feeding my daughter immediately as well. I told her actually I didn't need it. I was feeling a lot better, had my vision back, and the headache was gone. She still insisted I take the medicine and seemed to be triggered because of my refusal.

She then stated I needed to sign documentation saying I am refusing because based off of my serious diagnosis I could lose my vision or even my life and she didn't want to be held liable. Funny, if she was that concerned about my life and vision why didn't she try to help me sooner when I told her three weeks prior I thought I would die? She started going on saying that she's the only one who seems to be concerned about my health and she's only concerned about my vision, implying I wasn't taking my health seriously. Now this triggered me!

I asked her if she was so concerned about my health and particularly my vision why would she prescribe me cortical steroids indefinitely because studies show long-term usage have direct links to the development of cataracts! She may have been trying to "save" my vision at the moment, but what about the long-term effects?

I told her that I changed my diet, eliminating meat and all other animal byproducts, and she suggested I try to re-intro-duce meat into my diet and see what would happen because there's no way that was the actual reason. At that point I thought she was a quack and took her advice as a threat to my life and exited her office immediately. After all I've been through, re-introducing meat sounded asinine.

Chapter 3
How Food Affects the Body

America, the land of the free, a coveted nation where many desire to come and live out the American Dream. Full of prosperity and hope. However, the standard diet of this land of the free is destroying the health of many of its citizens. The Standard American Diet (SAD) is a modern dietary pattern afflicting American adults and children across the United States with long-term, damaging health consequences.

By definition, the Standard American Diet consists of ultra-processed foods, added sugar, fat, and sodium. Consumption of fruits, vegetables, whole grains, legumes, and lean protein is greatly lacking in this diet.

What does the Standard American Diet consist of?

- Fried foods
- Grain-based desserts
- High-fat dairy
- Processed foods

- Processed meats (e.g., bacon and deli meats)
- Red meat
- Refined grains (e.g., white pasta, white flour, etc.)
- Sugar-sweetened beverages

Besides all the fried, processed, high-fat, high-sugary foods that make up the Standard American Diet, Americans consume significantly more meat and meat products than most countries in the world. Meat consumption in the United States has nearly doubled in the last century. Americans are now among the top per capita meat consumers in the world; the average American eats more than three times the global average.

A growing body of evidence suggests Americans' taste for meat and animal products is putting them at greater risk for a range of health problems.

What does this type of diet do to the human body? The over-indulging doesn't come without consequence. As a result, nearly half of American adults suffer from one or more chronic illnesses that are related to poor dietary choices. The result of these choices is a build-up of mucus, fat, phlegm, or plaque throughout various areas of the body, causing disease.

Dr. Sebi also believed that all disease stemmed from mucus and the solution to curing disease was to rid the body of all excess mucus. Today, nearly 40% of U.S. adults are considered obese, which contributes to an upward trend of chronic illness.

To name a few implications you can face as a result of eating this way: cancer, cardiovascular disease, higher fasting blood glucose, hypertension, increased LDL cholesterol, Type 2 diabetes, and as discussed before, autoimmune diseases.

So what exactly did I eat in those two weeks? I went on a raw vegan diet for the first week, consuming only raw fruits, vegetables, and nuts. The second week I introduced cooked vegan dishes, limiting potato, rice, and absolutely no bread or other gluten products. Instead, I used quinoa, spelt flour, and millet.

Every day I took flaxseed oil, a colon cleansing supplement, and a vision-boosting supplement, all given to me by Dr. C. That was all I did as far as my diet was concerned to regain my vision. A very simple and all-natural method without harsh medications or hospitalization. It was a complete reset of my immune system and various bodily functions.

Dr. C also instructed that I stay away from all cooking oils. Canola oil, vegetable oil, corn oil, sunflower oil were all off limits. These oils do not digest well in the body, instead solidifying and forming these areas of plaque and mucus build-up which I was avoiding. The only oils I used were olive, coconut, grape seed, avocado, and flaxseed oil.

Eating this diet of "clean" foods helped to flush my system and jump-start my immune system reset.

Chapter 4
Detoxing the Body

I remember growing up, my Jamaican grandmother would give us something called a "washout" every few months. It was an herbal mixture with a horrible taste that did exactly what it was named to do: wash you out. We took these during times, usually the weekends, when we knew we didn't have to go outside for at least two days. We did this because if you did, you would face sheer embarrassment. The washout cleans out your body thoroughly through excretion, and you would have "the runs" for at least two days. When the washout was finished with your body, you would feel lighter and emptier.

Well, this is also what I did for two weeks while I was restoring my vision. As I was eating clean, I was also detoxing my body with all-natural supplements and washing out all the mess I'd accumulated over the years.

The Science of Detoxification

Detoxification is more than just a trendy health concept—it's a critical biological process that helps our body maintain optimal functioning. At its core, detoxification means cleansing the blood by removing impurities through the body's primary elimination systems. These include the liver, kidneys, intestines, lungs, lymphatic system, and skin.

The liver plays a central role in this process. It acts like a sophisticated filter, processing toxins and transforming them into less harmful substances that can be safely eliminated from the body. Think of it as your body's own waste management system, working tirelessly to protect you from harmful substances accumulated through diet, environment, and lifestyle.

Types of Toxins We Accumulate

- Environmental pollutants
- Processed food chemicals
- Excess hormones
- Metabolic waste products
- Heavy metals
- Preservatives and artificial additives

Why Regular Detoxification Matters

The Standard American Diet, laden with processed foods, chemicals, and artificial ingredients, constantly burdens our body's detoxification systems. Over time, this can lead to:

- Reduced organ efficiency

- Compromised immune function
- Increased inflammation
- Metabolic disruptions
- Potential chronic health issues

Experts suggest detoxing at least four times a year to help reset and support your body's natural cleansing mechanisms. When your organs are free of accumulated toxins, they can function more efficiently, effectively keeping essential nutrients while eliminating waste.

My Personal Detox Journey

During my two-week healing process, I embraced a comprehensive detoxification approach. I used natural supplements designed to support the body's elimination systems, combined with a strict vegan diet that minimized toxin intake while providing nutrient-dense foods to support cellular health.

The result? Not just a cleansing of my physical body, but a complete reset of my immune system and bodily functions. By removing processed foods, harmful oils, and introducing clean, whole foods, I gave my body the opportunity to heal and regenerate.

Practical Detoxification Strategies

- Stay hydrated with pure water
- Consume foods rich in antioxidants
- Minimize processed food intake
- Support liver health with cruciferous vegetables
- Practice periodic fasting or cleansing
- Reduce exposure to environmental toxins

- Incorporate herbal supplements that support detoxification

While my grandmother's "washout" might have seemed extreme, it embodied a traditional wisdom about periodic body cleansing that modern science is now beginning to validate. Detoxification isn't about a quick fix, but a holistic approach to maintaining long-term health and preventing chronic diseases.

Chapter 5
Supplemental Nutrition

After clearing out your body with a detox, it's essential to build it back up to proper nutrition. One way to obtain that nutrition is through the food you eat, and another way is with supplements. These add in any vitamins or minerals that may be lacking in your diet and keep your body in optimal health.

Common supplements include:

- Vitamins (multivitamins or individual vitamins like vitamin D and biotin)
- Minerals (calcium, magnesium, iron)
- Botanicals or herbs (echinacea, ginger)

Supplements target deficiencies in the body and specific organs. If an organ isn't operating at its optimal performance, it may be lacking certain minerals or vitamins. For example, you can take supplements that support:

- Heart health
- Eye function
- Kidney support
- Liver function

During my detox and cleanse, I was given three types of supplements: flaxseed oil, a colon cleansing supplement, and an eye and brain support supplement. I learned how beneficial flaxseed was for the detoxing process and your overall immune health, especially in combating multiple sclerosis and other autoimmune diseases.

Flaxseed Oil: A Nutritional Powerhouse

Flaxseed oil offers several potential benefits for immunity:

1. Rich in omega-3 fatty acids that reduce inflammation
2. Anti-inflammatory properties that modulate immune response
3. Antioxidants that neutralize harmful free radicals
4. Prebiotic support for gut health
5. Essential nutrients supporting immune function
6. Improved skin health as a protective barrier

The Crucial Role of Colon Health

The colon plays a significant role in immune function:

1. Houses the gut microbiome, critical for immune response
2. Produces immunoglobulins (antibodies)
3. Helps the immune system distinguish between harmless and harmful substances

4. Provides mucosal immunity
5. Regulates body-wide inflammation
6. Produces beneficial short-chain fatty acids

Discovering Papaya Seeds: A Natural Supplement

During my recent travels to Ghana, I discovered the incredible health benefits of papaya seeds. These powerful natural supplements offer numerous health advantages:

- Powerful antioxidant properties
- Supports gut health
- Aids in weight loss
- Lowers cholesterol
- Potential anti-cancer properties
- Protects kidney and heart health
- Reduces inflammation
- Supports skin health
- Antibacterial properties
- Helps manage menstrual issues
- Supports liver health
- Assists in food poisoning prevention

However, it's crucial to use papaya seeds cautiously:

- Consume no more than one teaspoon daily
- Avoid if pregnant or breastfeeding
- May impact male fertility

For comprehensive immune system support in fighting autoimmune diseases, I recommend incorporating flaxseed oil and papaya seed supplements into your nutrition plan.

Disclaimer: Always consult with a healthcare professional before starting any new supplement regimen.

Chapter 6
Mindful Mindset and Healing

Besides diet, if you recall from a previous chapter, I shared my story about the toxic relationship I was in at the time of my blindness. Along with the physical toll, the mental and spiritual toxicity that surrounded me played a major part in my declining health. Not only was the relationship physically abusive, but the mental abuse was even more harmful. It deeply affected my self-esteem, how I viewed myself, and how I spoke to myself, both inwardly and outwardly. I began to believe negative things about myself—feelings of worthlessness and hopelessness plagued my mind. The constant stress of these battles only worsened the pain.

But it wasn't just in that moment of my life when this toxic mindset held me captive. It was something I had battled my entire life. Childhood traumas had manifested into a negative self-image and a tendency to stay in unfulfilling, codependent relationships. That relationship, which had lasted for ten years, had reached its breaking point, and the chaos was at an all-time high. I realized that the pain from my headaches would triple in intensity during arguments, and I had no choice but to disengage completely. As soon as I stepped away and took a deep breath, the pain would subside. I learned to walk away, becoming intentionally "blind, mute, and deaf" when provoked into arguments. This is when I truly began to understand the importance of meditation— clearing the mind and blocking out all external distractions. You often hear about the benefits of meditation, but to actually practice it during your toughest times is a whole different experience.

Sometimes, even without provocation, the headaches would escalate. The pain was so severe that I felt certain death was near. It was excruciating. But whenever thoughts of death crossed my mind, I would think of my one-year-old daughter. Who would raise her? Who would love her the way only I could? It was in that moment that I found my strength. When death entered my mind, I spoke out loud, confronting it: "I will not die! I will live! I will see her grow up. I will help her in her times of need. I will raise her to the best of my ability!" It might have seemed crazy, but it worked like a charm. In that moment, I realized the power of my words and started to free myself from mental slavery.

I became hyper-aware of the words I allowed to leave my mouth and develop in my mind. Negative emotions and self-talk only led to more negativity and pain. But positive self-talk, affirming myself, and embracing positive energy resulted in less pain and more power. Just 12 days after losing my vision and starting my wellness journey, I regained my eyesight—shocking doctors, family, friends, and even my toxic ex. I had a completely new outlook on life. It became a priority to surround myself with people who uplifted me, showed me love, and reciprocated respect.

But my journey to mental health didn't end there. Healing—mentally, emotionally, and spiritually—takes time. In addition to distancing myself from toxic relationships, I had to work inward to understand why I ever allowed them to affect me. It was actually my search for relief from physical and emotional pain that led me to a career in Massage Therapy. That's where I started to understand how trapped emotions could manifest as physical pain in the body.

While in massage school, during a session with another student, I experienced what is called an "emotional release." This is a phenomenon in massage therapy where a person's emotional pain is stored in a particular area of their body. When that area is worked on, the person often cries as they experience the release of that pain. For me, it happened around my hips. The release was painful, but it felt so good at the same time. And in that moment, I began to cry, transported back to the trauma that had caused the pain. I realized I had been holding onto that pain for years. From that point on, I made it my mission to confront my traumas, understand them, and release them.

I've learned since then that nothing in life is left to chance—there are no coincidences. Life has proven this to me time and time again. It was these circumstances that deepened my commitment to healing my mind, body, and spirit. I opened a business called The Wellness House of Healing and began hosting community events in The Bronx, all in pursuit of healing for myself and others. During one of those events, I learned from a colleague about Shadow Work and healing the Inner Child.

Shadow Work involves working with your unconscious mind to uncover parts of yourself that you repress or hide. This may include trauma or aspects of your personality you subconsciously deem undesirable. Healing your Inner Child is about nurturing the part of you that may have been neglected in childhood. It's about reconnecting with your true self, understanding how early experiences shaped your personality and how you perceive the world today. Often, healing your Inner Child involves confronting it, offering love, security, and reassurance so that the adult subconscious can finally be free. These are deep, difficult subjects, but if you feel you're in need of therapy, I recommend starting with these areas. Your heart and spirit will thank you for it later.

The road to healing is neither quick nor easy. In fact, it can be brutal, ugly, and painful. It takes time, patience, reflection, and a great deal of love and tenderness to reach the other side. But what awaits you is the pure beauty of self-love. So be gentle with yourself. Be kind, be brave, and take the necessary steps toward self-healing.

Chapter 7
Seven Years Later
Staying Disease Free

It has now been seven years since my first and only MS diagnosis, and I am happy and proud to say that I am still disease-free. Ironically, as I began writing this book, I started experiencing feelings similar to those I had seven years ago. I firmly believe—or rather, I know—that a higher power and universal elements are at play, and I have no doubt this was not a coincidence. It served as a reminder of all I've been through, helping me to guide every reader of this book on ways to combat Multiple Sclerosis and other autoimmune diseases.

When I first started my cleanse seven years ago, I committed to a vegan lifestyle for eight months. Losing my vision was the biggest scare of my life, and I was determined to never experience that again. During this time, I focused on preparing nutrient-dense meals, like green smoothies packed with kale, spinach, and fruits, and hearty salads with quinoa, avocados, and a variety of fresh vegetables. I also incorporated herbal teas and plenty of water to support detoxification.

Supplements, such as vitamin D, B12, and omega-3s, were key elements in my routine.

Eventually, however, I started eating meat again. Crazy, right? Hey, I'm only human! Yet, I'm still disease-free. Why is that? My theory is that the long period of detoxing had lasting effects. Even after reintroducing meat into my diet, I continued periodic cleanses every few months to maintain balance. These cleanses would often include juice fasting, reducing processed foods, and focusing on mindfulness to realign my body and mind.

That said, after the birth of my middle child 3½ years ago, I struggled to keep up with those periodic cleanses. I believe that's why I started to feel symptoms again as I began writing this book. Recognizing this, I decided to take two weeks off for a mental and physical cleanse, and now I'm free of symptoms again. In fact, I'm planning to return to a strict alkaline diet very soon to maintain optimal health. This diet will focus on high-alkaline foods like leafy greens, cucumbers, bell peppers, and lemons, while avoiding acidic triggers like processed sugars, caffeine, and dairy.

Life is a journey, full of ups and downs, lessons, and growth. Embrace the ride, because you can't go back. It's only forward from here. Every day, make choices that help you be brave, happy, and healthy.

If you are experiencing symptoms or have been diagnosed with MS or any autoimmune disease, I highly recommend trying a cleanse, nutritional supplementation, and mental clarification. You have absolutely nothing to lose and everything to gain. You might reclaim your life in ways you never imagined. To support your journey, consider starting with small steps: experiment with simple, plant-based meals, journal your thoughts to reduce stress, or try guided meditations to strengthen your mindset. Your body, mind, and spirit will thank you, and I'm confident you'll experience positive, life-changing results.

38

Resources For Your Journey
Grocery List for Your Autoimmune Reset

Fruits

- Apples
- Bananas (small or burro bananas, not Cavendish)
- Berries (strawberries, blueberries, blackberries, raspberries, elderberries)
- Cherries
- Dates (unsulfured, natural)
- Figs (fresh or dried)
- Grapes (seeded, preferably dark-skinned)
- Limes (with seeds)
- Mangoes
- Melons (cantaloupe, honeydew, watermelon with seeds)
- Oranges (Seville or sour)
- Papayas
- Peaches
- Pears

- Plums
- Prickly pear (cactus fruit)
- Soursop

Vegetables

- Amaranth greens
- Bell peppers
- Cactus (Nopales)
- Cucumbers
- Dandelion greens
- Kale
- Lettuce (e.g., romaine, butter, or mixed greens)
- Mushrooms (oyster, portobello)
- Okra
- Onions (purple preferred)
- Seaweed (wakame, nori, dulse)
- Squash (zucchini, butternut, acorn)
- Tomatoes (cherry and plum varieties only)
- Watercress
- Zucchini

Grains & Flours

- Amaranth
- Fonio
- Kamut
- Quinoa
- Rye
- Spelt
- Teff
- Wild rice

Legumes (Minimal)

- Chickpeas (garbanzo beans)
- Lentils

Nuts & Seeds

- Brazil nuts
- Hemp seeds
- Sesame seeds
- Walnuts
- Raw almond butter (if allowed)

Herbs & Seasonings

- Basil
- Bay leaf
- Cilantro
- Dill
- Oregano
- Sage
- Thyme
- Cayenne pepper
- Pure sea salt
- Onion powder
- Red pepper flakes

Oils

- Coconut oil (unrefined, cold-pressed)
- Olive oil (extra virgin, cold-pressed)

- Avocado oil

Sweeteners

- Date sugar
- Pure agave syrup

Seaweed & Algae

- Irish moss
- Bladderwrack
- Dulse flakes

7 Day Autoimmune Reset Meal Plan

Week 1

Day 1

Breakfast: Soursop smoothie (soursop, seeded grapes, dates, and spring water).

Snack: Fresh figs or an apple.

Lunch: Large kale and arugula salad with sliced cucumbers, cherry tomatoes, avocado, red onion, and olive oil + lime dressing.

Dinner: Zucchini noodles with cherry tomato and bell pepper sauce, seasoned with fresh basil and oregano.

Day 2

Breakfast: Chia pudding (made with coconut milk, date sugar, and topped with fresh blueberries).

Snack: Handful of Brazil nuts.

Lunch: Quinoa bowl with sautéed okra, mushrooms, and onions, drizzled with olive oil and lime juice.

Dinner: Stuffed bell peppers with wild rice, chickpeas, diced tomatoes, and herbs (baked).

Day 3

Breakfast: Mango and papaya fruit bowl topped with hemp seeds and shredded coconut.

Snack: A handful of walnuts and dried figs.

Lunch: Spelt tortillas stuffed with sautéed amaranth greens, avocado, and sliced cucumbers.

Dinner: Butternut squash soup with a side of watercress salad and olive oil dressing.

Day 4

Breakfast: Smoothie with burro bananas, seeded grapes, and coconut water.

Snack: Cucumber slices with sea salt and a squeeze of lime.

Lunch: Wild rice salad with diced tomatoes, cucumbers, and a light olive oil + cayenne pepper dressing.

Dinner: Grilled zucchini slices with a chickpea and tomato stew.

Day 5

Breakfast: Date and fig smoothie with coconut milk.

Snack: Fresh cherries.

Lunch: Spelt pasta with homemade cherry tomato sauce, topped with fresh basil.

Dinner: Sautéed mushrooms, onions, and kale with quinoa on the side.

Day 6

Breakfast: Watermelon slices and a side of wild blueberries.

Snack: Handful of sesame seeds and dried dates.

Lunch: Cucumber and avocado gazpacho with a side of dandelion greens salad.

Dinner: Grilled portobello mushrooms stuffed with wild rice, chickpeas, and diced bell peppers.

Day 7

Breakfast: Fresh papaya bowl topped with hemp seeds and coconut flakes.

Snack: A handful of walnuts and a sliced apple.

Lunch: Quinoa and arugula salad with diced tomatoes, cucumbers, and olive oil dressing.

Dinner: Zucchini noodles tossed in a creamy avocado and basil sauce with a side of sautéed mushrooms.

Week 2

Day 8

Breakfast: Smoothie with burro bananas, dates, and coconut water.

Snack: Dried figs and Brazil nuts.

Lunch: Kamut flatbread with mashed avocado, sliced cucumber, and arugula.

Dinner: Spelt and chickpea stew with diced tomatoes, onions, and cayenne pepper.

Day 9

Breakfast: Fresh mango slices with a side of seeded grapes.

Snack: A handful of sesame seeds.

Lunch: Watercress and kale salad with avocado, cherry tomatoes, and lime-olive oil dressing.

Dinner: Grilled zucchini boats stuffed with quinoa, mushrooms, and tomatoes.

Day 10

Breakfast: Chia pudding with coconut milk, date sugar, and topped with fresh strawberries.

Snack: Fresh cherries or an apple.

Lunch: Wild rice bowl with sautéed onions, okra, and bell peppers.

Dinner: Butternut squash soup with a side of spelt flatbread.

Day 11

Breakfast: Papaya smoothie with coconut water and lime.

Snack: A handful of walnuts and dried dates.

Lunch: Zucchini noodles with avocado pesto sauce and a side of watercress salad.

Dinner: Portobello mushrooms stuffed with chickpeas, wild rice, and tomatoes.

Day 12

Breakfast: Burro bananas and fresh blueberries.

Snack: Cucumber slices with lime and sea salt.

Lunch: Quinoa and dandelion greens salad with olive oil and cayenne dressing.

Dinner: Spelt pasta with cherry tomato sauce and sautéed mushrooms.

Day 13

Breakfast: Watermelon and mango fruit bowl.

Snack: A handful of Brazil nuts and dried figs.

Lunch: Kamut flatbread with avocado, arugula, and cucumber slices.

Dinner: Chickpea and vegetable stew with butternut squash.

Day 14

Breakfast: Smoothie with seeded grapes, figs, and coconut water.

Snack: Fresh cherries or an apple.

Lunch: Arugula and kale salad with avocado, tomatoes, and olive oil dressing.

Dinner: Wild rice with sautéed mushrooms, onions, and bell peppers.

20 Delicious Raw and Cooked Vegan Meals for Reset

1. Soursop Smoothie

Ingredients:

- 1 cup soursop pulp (seeded)
- 1 cup seeded grapes
- 3 dates (pitted)
- 1 cup spring water

Instructions:

1. Blend all ingredients in a blender until smooth.
2. Serve immediately and enjoy!

2. Kale & Arugula Salad with Avocado Lime Dressing

Ingredients:

- 2 cups kale (chopped, stems removed)

- 2 cups arugula
- 1 cucumber (sliced)
- 1 avocado (diced)
- 1/2 red onion (thinly sliced)
- 1/2 cup cherry tomatoes (halved)
- 1 lime (juiced)
- 2 tbsp extra virgin olive oil
- Sea salt to taste

Instructions:

1. In a large bowl, combine kale, arugula, cucumber, red onion, and cherry tomatoes.
2. Toss with lime juice, olive oil, and sea salt.
3. Top with diced avocado and serve.

3. Zucchini Noodles with Avocado Basil Sauce

Ingredients:

- 2 zucchinis (spiralized into noodles)
- 1 avocado
- 1/4 cup fresh basil leaves
- 1 garlic clove
- 2 tbsp olive oil
- 1/2 lime (juiced)
- Sea salt to taste

Instructions:

1. Blend avocado, basil, garlic, olive oil, lime juice, and salt until creamy.

2. Toss zucchini noodles with the sauce until evenly coated.
3. Serve fresh.

4. Wild Rice Salad

Ingredients:

- 1 cup cooked wild rice
- 1/2 cup cherry tomatoes (halved)
- 1/2 cucumber (diced)
- 2 tbsp red onion (minced)
- 2 tbsp olive oil
- 1 tbsp lime juice
- 1/4 tsp cayenne pepper
- Sea salt to taste

Instructions:

1. In a bowl, combine wild rice, cherry tomatoes, cucumber, and red onion.
2. Drizzle with olive oil and lime juice.
3. Sprinkle cayenne pepper and sea salt, then toss to combine.

5. Chia Pudding with Coconut Milk

Ingredients:

- 1/4 cup chia seeds
- 1 cup coconut milk
- 1 tbsp date sugar
- 1/2 cup fresh blueberries

Instructions:

1. Mix chia seeds, coconut milk, and date sugar in a jar. Let sit for 2–3 hours or overnight.
2. Top with fresh blueberries before serving.

6. Butternut Squash Soup

Ingredients:

- 2 cups butternut squash (cubed)
- 1/2 onion (diced)
- 2 tbsp olive oil
- 2 cups spring water
- 1/2 tsp cayenne pepper
- Sea salt to taste

Instructions:

1. Sauté onions in olive oil until translucent.
2. Add butternut squash and cook for 5 minutes.
3. Add spring water, bring to a boil, then simmer until squash is tender.
4. Blend until smooth. Season with cayenne pepper and salt.

7. Grilled Zucchini Boats

Ingredients:

- 2 zucchinis (halved lengthwise, seeds scooped out)
- 1 cup cooked quinoa
- 1/2 cup cherry tomatoes (diced)

- 1/4 cup red onion (diced)
- 2 tbsp olive oil
- 1/4 tsp oregano
- Sea salt to taste

Instructions:

1. Brush zucchini halves with olive oil and season with salt.
2. Grill zucchini until tender.
3. Mix quinoa, tomatoes, onion, oregano, and olive oil in a bowl.
4. Fill zucchini boats with the mixture and serve.

8. Spelt Tortillas with Avocado & Greens

Ingredients:

- 2 spelt tortillas
- 1 avocado (mashed)
- 1/2 cucumber (sliced)
- 1 cup arugula

Instructions:

1. Spread mashed avocado over spelt tortillas.
2. Layer with cucumber slices and arugula.
3. Roll up and enjoy!

9. Mango & Papaya Fruit Bowl

Ingredients:

- 1 mango (diced)
- 1/2 papaya (diced)
- 1 tbsp hemp seeds
- 1 tbsp shredded coconut

Instructions:

1. Combine mango and papaya in a bowl.
2. Sprinkle with hemp seeds and shredded coconut.

10. Stuffed Bell Peppers

Ingredients:

- 2 bell peppers (halved, seeds removed)
- 1 cup cooked wild rice
- 1/2 cup chickpeas
- 1/4 cup cherry tomatoes (diced)
- 1/4 cup onion (diced)
- 1 tbsp olive oil
- 1/4 tsp thyme
- Sea salt to taste

Instructions:

1. Preheat oven to 375°F (if baking).
2. Mix wild rice, chickpeas, tomatoes, onion, olive oil, thyme, and salt in a bowl.
3. Fill bell pepper halves with the mixture.
4. Bake for 20 minutes or enjoy raw if preferred.

Caribbean Inspired

11. Plantain & Coconut Breakfast Bowl

Ingredients:

- 1 burro banana (sliced)
- 1/2 cup coconut milk
- 1 tbsp shredded coconut
- 1 tbsp hemp seeds
- 1 tbsp date sugar

Instructions:

1. Heat coconut milk until warm (if desired).
2. Add sliced burro banana to a bowl and pour coconut milk over it.
3. Top with shredded coconut, hemp seeds, and date sugar.

12. Mango Lime Salsa

Ingredients:

- 1 mango (diced)
- 1/2 cucumber (diced)
- 1/4 red onion (minced)
- 1 lime (juiced)
- 1 tbsp cilantro (chopped)
- Sea salt to taste

Instructions:

1. Combine all ingredients in a bowl and mix well.
2. Serve as a dip with raw veggie chips or as a topping for zucchini noodles or salads.

13. Callaloo-Inspired Greens Sauté

Ingredients:

- 2 cups amaranth greens or kale (chopped)
- 1/2 onion (sliced)
- 1/2 red bell pepper (sliced)
- 2 tbsp olive oil
- 1/4 tsp thyme
- Sea salt to taste

Instructions:

1. Heat olive oil in a pan and sauté onion and bell pepper until soft.
2. Add greens, thyme, and sea salt, cooking until wilted.
3. Serve with wild rice or quinoa.

14. Ackee-Style Mushrooms

Ingredients:

- 1 cup oyster mushrooms (torn into pieces)
- 1/2 onion (sliced)
- 1/2 red bell pepper (sliced)
- 1 garlic clove (minced)
- 2 tbsp olive oil
- 1/4 tsp thyme
- Sea salt to taste

Instructions:

1. Heat olive oil in a pan and sauté onion, garlic, and bell pepper until fragrant.
2. Add mushrooms, thyme, and sea salt. Cook until mushrooms are tender.
3. Serve with spelt flatbread or quinoa.

15. Spicy Coconut Okra Soup

Ingredients:

- 1 cup okra (sliced)
- 1/2 onion (diced)
- 1/2 cup coconut milk
- 2 cups spring water
- 1/4 tsp cayenne pepper
- 1/4 tsp thyme
- Sea salt to taste

Instructions:

1. Sauté onion in olive oil until soft.
2. Add okra, coconut milk, spring water, cayenne, thyme, and sea salt. Simmer until okra is tender.

16. Coconut Lime Wild Rice

Ingredients:

- 1 cup cooked wild rice
- 1/4 cup coconut milk
- 1 lime (juiced)

- 1 tbsp cilantro (chopped)
- Sea salt to taste

Instructions:

1. Mix cooked wild rice with coconut milk, lime juice, and sea salt.
2. Garnish with chopped cilantro before serving.

17. Jerk-Style Grilled Vegetables

Ingredients:

- 1 zucchini (sliced)
- 1 bell pepper (sliced)
- 1/2 onion (sliced)
- 2 tbsp olive oil
- 1/2 tsp cayenne pepper
- 1/2 tsp thyme
- 1/2 tsp onion powder
- Sea salt to taste

Instructions:

1. Mix olive oil, cayenne pepper, thyme, onion powder, and sea salt in a bowl.
2. Toss vegetables in the mixture.
3. Grill or roast until tender.

18. Tamarind Dressing

Ingredients:

- 2 tbsp tamarind paste
- 1 tbsp olive oil
- 1 tbsp date sugar
- 1/2 lime (juiced)
- 1/4 tsp cayenne pepper

Instructions:

1. Whisk all ingredients together in a bowl.
2. Use as a salad dressing or drizzle over roasted veggies.

19. Caribbean Coconut Curry with Chickpeas

Ingredients:

- 1 cup cooked chickpeas
- 1/2 onion (diced)
- 1/2 red bell pepper (sliced)
- 1/2 cup coconut milk
- 1/4 tsp curry powder (homemade or alkaline)
- 1 tbsp olive oil
- Sea salt to taste

Instructions:

1. Sauté onion and bell pepper in olive oil until soft.
2. Add chickpeas, coconut milk, curry powder, and sea salt.
3. Simmer for 10 minutes and serve with wild rice or quinoa.

20. Spelt Festival (Fried Dough)

Ingredients:

- 1 cup spelt flour
- 1 tbsp date sugar
- 1/4 tsp sea salt
- 1/4 cup coconut milk
- 1 tbsp coconut oil

Instructions:

1. Mix spelt flour, date sugar, and sea salt in a bowl. Slowly add coconut milk to form a dough.
2. Roll small pieces into oblong shapes.
3. Heat coconut oil in a pan and fry dough pieces until golden brown.

Ghanaian Inspired

1. Alkaline Jollof Rice

Ingredients:

- 1 cup wild rice (cooked)
- 1/2 cup cherry tomatoes (blended into a sauce)
- 1/2 red bell pepper (blended)
- 1/2 onion (diced)
- 1/4 tsp cayenne pepper
- 1/4 tsp thyme
- 2 tbsp olive oil
- Sea salt to taste

Instructions:

1. Sauté diced onions in olive oil until soft.
2. Add blended tomatoes and bell pepper. Simmer for 10 minutes.
3. Season with cayenne, thyme, and sea salt. Add cooked wild rice and mix well.
4. Cook on low heat for 5 minutes and serve.

2. Waakye-Inspired Wild Rice and Chickpeas

Ingredients:

- 1 cup cooked wild rice
- 1/2 cup cooked chickpeas
- 1/2 onion (sliced)
- 1/4 tsp cayenne pepper
- 2 tbsp olive oil
- 1 tsp dandelion greens (optional, for "waakye leaves" flavor)
- Sea salt to taste

Instructions:

1. Heat olive oil in a pan and sauté onions until soft.
2. Add chickpeas, cooked wild rice, cayenne, and dandelion greens.
3. Stir-fry for 5 minutes, season with sea salt, and serve warm.

3. Yam Substitute: Fried Burro Plantains

Ingredients:

- 2 burro bananas (ripe, sliced diagonally)
- 2 tbsp coconut oil
- Sea salt to taste

Instructions:

1. Heat coconut oil in a frying pan.
2. Fry burro banana slices until golden brown on both sides.
3. Sprinkle with a pinch of sea salt and serve as a side dish.

4. Light Soup with Vegetables

Ingredients:

- 2 cups cherry tomatoes (blended)
- 1/2 onion (blended)
- 1/2 red bell pepper (blended)
- 1 cup okra (sliced)
- 1/2 zucchini (cubed)
- 2 cups spring water
- 1/4 tsp cayenne pepper
- Sea salt to taste

Instructions:

1. Bring the blended tomato, onion, and bell pepper mix to a boil in spring water.

2. Add okra, zucchini, cayenne, and sea salt. Simmer until vegetables are tender.

5. Kenkey-Inspired Fermented Spelt Dumplings

Ingredients:

- 1 cup spelt flour
- 1/2 cup spring water
- 1/4 tsp sea salt

Instructions:

1. Mix spelt flour, water, and salt to form a dough. Let sit for 2 hours to lightly ferment.
2. Form small dough balls, then wrap them in banana leaves or parchment paper.
3. Steam for 20–30 minutes. Serve with spicy tomato salsa.

6. Garden Egg Stew (Eggplant Stew)

Ingredients:

- 1 cup eggplant (cubed)
- 1/2 cup cherry tomatoes (blended)
- 1/2 onion (diced)
- 1/4 tsp cayenne pepper
- 2 tbsp olive oil
- Sea salt to taste

Instructions:

1. Sauté onions in olive oil until translucent.
2. Add blended tomatoes, eggplant, cayenne, and sea salt. Cook until eggplant is tender.
3. Serve with wild rice or spelt flatbread.

7. Okra Stir-Fry with Wild Rice

Ingredients:

- 1 cup okra (sliced)
- 1/2 onion (sliced)
- 1/2 red bell pepper (sliced)
- 2 tbsp olive oil
- 1/4 tsp thyme
- Sea salt to taste

Instructions:

1. Heat olive oil in a pan and sauté onions and bell peppers.
2. Add okra, thyme, and sea salt. Cook until okra is tender but not slimy.
3. Serve over wild rice.

8. Spicy Coconut Soup

Ingredients:

- 1/2 cup coconut milk
- 2 cups spring water
- 1/2 onion (diced)
- 1/2 cup cherry tomatoes (blended)
- 1/4 tsp cayenne pepper

- 1/2 zucchini (cubed)
- Sea salt to taste

Instructions:

1. Sauté onions in a pot until soft.
2. Add blended tomatoes, coconut milk, water, cayenne, and zucchini.
3. Simmer until zucchini is tender.

9. Spelt Flatbread with Avocado Dip

Flatbread Ingredients:

- 1 cup spelt flour
- 1/4 cup spring water
- 1/4 tsp sea salt

Avocado Dip Ingredients:

- 1 avocado
- 1/2 lime (juiced)
- 1 tbsp olive oil
- Sea salt to taste

Instructions:

1. Mix spelt flour, water, and sea salt to form a dough. Roll out flat and cook on a hot skillet until golden on both sides.
2. Blend avocado, lime juice, olive oil, and sea salt until creamy.
3. Serve flatbread with the avocado dip.

10. Shito-Inspired Pepper Sauce

Ingredients:

- 1/2 cup cherry tomatoes (blended)
- 1/2 onion (diced)
- 1 garlic clove (minced)
- 2 tbsp olive oil
- 1/4 tsp cayenne pepper
- 1/4 tsp thyme
- Sea salt to taste

Instructions:

1. Heat olive oil in a pan and sauté onion and garlic until fragrant.
2. Add blended tomatoes, cayenne, thyme, and sea salt. Simmer for 10–15 minutes until thickened.
3. Serve as a spicy condiment for wild rice or flatbreads.

About the Author

Alycea K. Shirley is a Bronx Native, Licensed Massage Therapist and founder of The Wellness House of Healing. A Wellness Center, specializing in massage and herbal and holistic remedies. In 2016 she used her passion and knowledge in natural and holistic healing to ultimately save her vision and her very own life. She has traveled abroad to Ghana to further her studies of natural remedies, healings, and life experiences.

For more information, or to book an event, contact: Alyceashirley@gmail.com

Acknowledgments

Firstly, I would like to give all thanks and praise to The Most High, the source of my strength and abilities. Who has been there through all the obstacles, lessons, and highs and lows. Also, Dr. Sebi and his teachings on his unique diet of alkaline plant based electric food. Special thanks to Dr. C for his guidance and extraordinary knowledge. To my parents, who even when they didn't understand me, always still decided to support me in my decisions. My grandparents, who instilled a love for natural remedies in me. My children; Tiwa, Iman, and Boatemaa. They are the people in this realm who give me strength.